The Art & Chore of Cutting Nails

Scratched by

Zeeshan Mahmud

Why is it such a darn chore!

I feel you reader on that! It can definitely feel like a chore sometimes. Maybe it's because it's one of those tasks that feels like it constantly needs doing, kind of like laundry or dishes. Plus, it's a small task that requires attention to detail, and sometimes it's just hard to find the motivation for those little things.

For one, it's a task that requires some precision and care, especially if you want to avoid accidentally cutting too short or unevenly. Then there's the fact that it's a repetitive task that needs to be done regularly, adding to the feeling of monotony. Plus, some people might find it uncomfortable or even a bit gross, especially if they're not fond of the sensation or the sight of nail clippings. So, all those factors combined can definitely make it feel like a bit of a chore!

When you think about it, the return on investment for the time and effort spent cutting fingernails might not seem very high compared to other tasks. It's one of those things that you have to do for hygiene and grooming, but it doesn't necessarily bring the same immediate rewards or satisfaction as, say, completing a project or achieving a personal goal. It's kind of like maintenance work—it's necessary, but it's not always the most exciting or rewarding part of the day.But hey, think of it this way: after you're done, you'll have those satisfyingly trimmed nails ready for action!

History of nail-cutting

The history of cutting fingernails stretches back thousands of years and is intertwined with human culture and hygiene practices.
In ancient times, people used various methods to trim their nails, including biting them, using sharp stones, or cutting them with primitive tools like knives or scissors.

The methods varied depending on the culture and the available resources. For example, ancient Egyptians are believed to have used metal tools to trim their nails, while in ancient China, nail care was considered an important part of grooming, and intricate nail art was practiced. As civilizations progressed, so did nail care techniques. In ancient Rome, nail care became more sophisticated, with the use of metal tools specifically designed for trimming nails.

Similarly, in ancient India, nail care was considered an important aspect of personal hygiene, and special attention was paid to grooming nails as part of daily rituals. Throughout history, the perception of nail care has shifted, with nails often being associated with social status, hygiene, and even spiritual significance in some cultures. For example, in medieval Europe, long nails were sometimes seen as a sign of wealth and status, while in other cultures, trimmed nails were considered a symbol of cleanliness and purity.

Today, cutting fingernails is a common practice in cultures around the world, driven by hygiene, aesthetics, and personal grooming preferences. Modern nail care tools, such as nail clippers and manicure scissors, make the process easier and safer, and nail care has become an integral part of many people's daily routines.

Biting to cut?

Yes, biting nails to trim them is a common practice, although it's generally not recommended for a few reasons. When someone bites their nails, they're essentially using their teeth as makeshift scissors. While it might seem convenient, it can lead to several issues.

Firstly, biting nails can damage the nails themselves, causing them to become jagged, uneven, or even prone to infection if the skin around the nail bed is broken. It can also lead to issues with the teeth, such as chipping or wear, and potentially even dental problems if done frequently.

Additionally, nail biting is often associated with stress or anxiety, and it can become a habit that's difficult to break. People may find themselves biting their nails unconsciously, which can be frustrating.

Overall, while biting nails might seem like a quick fix, it's generally better to use proper nail care tools like clippers or scissors to trim them. These tools provide a more precise cut and are gentler on both the nails and the teeth.

DID YOU KNOW?

'Onychology' means the study of fingernails and toenails

Studies done?

Surveys and studies on personal grooming habits often highlight tasks like nail care as being perceived as tedious or mundane by many individuals. For example, a survey conducted by a personal care company might find that a significant portion of respondents consider nail care to be one of their least favorite grooming tasks. Additionally, research on habits and behaviors related to hygiene and self-care may provide insights into people's attitudes towards tasks like cutting fingernails. Studies on habits related to personal grooming, such as frequency of nail trimming or attitudes towards nail care products, may indirectly reflect people's feelings about the task itself.

Billion dollar industry!

The manicure and pedicure industry is indeed a significant and thriving sector within the beauty and personal care industry. It encompasses a wide range of services, from basic nail care and grooming to more elaborate treatments like nail art, gel manicures, and spa-style pedicures.

The industry generates billions of dollars in revenue globally each year, driven by a variety of factors. One key factor is the increasing emphasis on personal grooming and self-care in modern society. Many people view manicures and pedicures as a way to pamper themselves, boost their confidence, and enhance their overall appearance.

Moreover, the popularity of nail trends, such as intricate designs, unique colors, and innovative techniques, has contributed to the growth of the industry. Social media platforms like Instagram and Pinterest have played a significant role in popularizing nail art and inspiring people to experiment with different styles.

Additionally, the availability of professional nail salons and nail care products has made manicures and pedicures more accessible to a broader range of consumers. Whether it's a quick touch-up at a local salon or an indulgent spa day, there are options to suit every budget and preference.

Nail Care in Ancient Civilizations: A Glimpse into Ancient Nail Clipping Practices

The practice of nail care holds a significant place, serving as a testament to our ancestors' commitment to personal grooming and hygiene. Across ancient civilizations, from the majestic realms of Egypt to the vibrant cultures of Mesopotamia, nail care was not merely a mundane task but a ritualistic practice deeply embedded in social customs and religious beliefs.

Ancient Egypt

In the land of the Pharaohs, where grandeur and sophistication intertwined, nail care was elevated to an art form. Ancient Egyptians meticulously groomed their nails using an array of tools crafted from copper or bronze. Hieroglyphic inscriptions and archaeological findings reveal the meticulous attention paid to nail care, particularly among the elite classes and royalty. Delicate metal implements, resembling modern-day nail clippers in rudimentary form, were used to trim and shape the nails with precision, reflecting the Egyptians' mastery of craftsmanship and aesthetics.

Mesopotamia and the Fertile Crescent

In the cradle of civilization, amidst the fertile plains of Mesopotamia, nail care practices flourished alongside advancements in agriculture and urbanization. Sumerians and Babylonians, renowned for their ingenuity and cultural sophistication, practiced nail care as part of daily grooming rituals. Archaeological excavations unearthed clay tablets depicting scenes of manicured hands adorned with intricate nail art, indicating the significance of nail care in Mesopotamian society. While the specific tools used for nail clipping remain elusive, ancient texts and artifacts provide tantalizing glimpses into the meticulous grooming habits of these ancient peoples.

Indus Valley Civilization:

Nail care was woven into the fabric of everyday life during Indus Valley Civ. The inhabitants of the Indus Valley Civilization, known for their urban planning and sophisticated drainage systems, also exhibited a keen sense of personal hygiene. Archaeological discoveries, such as terracotta figurines depicting meticulously groomed individuals, suggest that nail care was an integral aspect of grooming practices in ancient India. While the precise methods of nail clipping remain speculative, the artifacts unearthed from Harappan sites offer tantalizing clues to the nail care practices of this enigmatic civilization.

Longest nails ever

The record for the longest fingernails ever on a human belongs to Lee Redmond from the United States. She held this record in the Guinness World Records until 2009. Redmond's nails had a combined length of 8.65 meters (28 feet 4.5 inches), with her longest nail, her right thumb, reaching an astonishing length of 0.6 meters (2 feet). She began growing her nails in 1979 and diligently maintained them for decades. However, tragically, she lost her record-setting nails in a car accident in 2009. Since then, the record for the longest fingernails on a pair of hands has been held by Ayanna Williams from the United States. Her nails measured a combined length of over 7 meters (24 feet).

Ritual of cutting nails

The ritual of cutting nails varies across cultures and often holds significance beyond mere hygiene. Here's a glimpse into how different cultures approach this practice:

East Asian Cultures: In countries like China, Japan, and Korea, there are traditional beliefs associated with nail-cutting. It's often considered unlucky to cut nails at night, as it's believed to bring bad luck or invite evil spirits. Some also believe that cutting nails on certain days of the week is more auspicious than others.

Indian Subcontinent: In India, Pakistan, Bangladesh, and neighboring countries, there are cultural and religious beliefs associated with nail-cutting. It's common for people to trim their nails on specific days, such as Saturdays or Tuesdays, while avoiding it on certain religious occasions or during mourning periods. Additionally, there's a tradition of burying or burning nail clippings to prevent negative energy or to avoid them being used for black magic.

Middle Eastern and Islamic Culture: In Islamic tradition, there's an emphasis on personal hygiene, including nail care. It's encouraged to keep nails clean and trimmed, with some scholars recommending nail-cutting at least every 40 days to maintain cleanliness. However, there aren't specific rituals associated with nail-cutting beyond the general emphasis on cleanliness in Islam.

Western Culture: In Western cultures, nail-cutting is primarily seen as a routine part of personal grooming and hygiene. There aren't typically any specific rituals or beliefs associated with it beyond maintaining cleanliness and aesthetics.

African Cultures: Practices surrounding nail-cutting vary widely across the diverse cultures of Africa. In some societies, there may be traditional rituals or taboos associated with nail care, while in others, it may simply be seen as a practical aspect of personal hygiene.

While the specifics may vary, the act of nail-cutting often carries symbolic significance related to cleanliness, health, and sometimes even spiritual beliefs across many cultures worldwide.

Superstition regarding nail-cutting

Superstitions surrounding nail-cutting exist in various cultures and often revolve around luck, health, and spiritual beliefs.

Luck and Fortune: In many cultures, there's a superstition that cutting nails at night brings bad luck or invites evil spirits into the home. This belief is particularly prevalent in East Asian cultures, where it's advised to avoid cutting nails after sunset.

Longevity: Some superstitions suggest that saving nail clippings and burying them can bring good luck or ensure a long life. This practice is found in cultures around the world, including parts of Asia and Africa.

Prevention of Black Magic: In some cultures, particularly in South Asia, there's a belief that nail clippings should be disposed of carefully to prevent them from being used for black magic or witchcraft. Burning or burying nail clippings is often recommended to ward off negative energy.

Health and Hygiene: Superstitions related to nail-cutting also extend to health and hygiene. For example, in some cultures, it's believed that cutting nails too short can lead to illness or cause injury to the fingers.

Avoiding Disputes: There's a superstition in some cultures that cutting nails on certain days, such as Sundays or Thursdays, can lead to arguments or disputes within the family. As a result, people may choose to avoid nail-cutting on these days to maintain harmony in the household.

While some may dismiss them as old wives' tales, they can still influence behavior and customs in many societies.

Nail art

Nail art is a creative form of self-expression that involves decorating fingernails and toenails with various designs, colors, and embellishments. It has become increasingly popular in recent years, evolving into a vibrant and diverse art form with countless possibilities for creativity.

Nail art can range from simple designs like solid colors or French tips to intricate patterns, geometric shapes, and elaborate motifs. It often incorporates techniques such as painting, stamping, stenciling, and freehand drawing using specialized nail art brushes and tools.

One of the appealing aspects of nail art is its versatility and adaptability to different styles and preferences. Whether someone prefers minimalist, understated designs or bold, eye-catching creations, there's something for everyone in the world of nail art.

Social media platforms like Instagram and Pinterest have played a significant role in popularizing nail art, providing a platform for nail artists to showcase their work and inspire others. Additionally, the availability of a wide range of nail polish colors, textures, and finishes has made it easier than ever for individuals to experiment with nail art at home or visit professional nail salons for customized designs.

Overall, nail art is a fun and creative way to express individuality, celebrate special occasions, or simply add a touch of flair to everyday life. With endless possibilities for design and decoration, it's no wonder that nail art has captured the imagination of people around the world.

Evolution of Nail Care: From Ancient Rituals to Modern Clippers

Nail care has been an essential aspect of personal grooming since ancient times, with civilizations around the world developing various techniques and tools for trimming and shaping nails. From the earliest civilizations to modern times, the practice of nail care has evolved, culminating in the invention of the modern nail clipper.

Ancient Nail Care Practices:

The history of nail care dates back thousands of years, with evidence of grooming practices found in archaeological sites from ancient civilizations. In ancient Egypt, for example, both men and women used metal tools made of copper or bronze to trim and shape their nails. Similarly, in ancient China and India, nail care was considered an important aspect of personal hygiene, with people using primitive tools like knives or sharp stones to groom their nails.

Medieval Innovations:

During the Middle Ages in Europe, nail care practices varied depending on social status and cultural norms. While some individuals, particularly nobility and royalty, may have had access to specialized grooming tools, the general population often relied on simple implements like knives or scissors to trim their nails. Hygiene practices during this time were generally less advanced, with nail care often being a practical necessity rather than a form of self-expression.

Rise of Modern Nail Clippers:

The invention of the modern nail clipper revolutionized nail care practices and made trimming nails significantly easier and safer. The precise origins of the nail clipper are unclear, but it is believed to have been developed in the late 19th or early 20th century. The design of the modern nail clipper consists of two levered blades that are pressed together to cut the nail cleanly and efficiently. The invention of the nail clipper represented a significant advancement in nail care technology, providing a safer and more convenient alternative to traditional grooming methods. Its compact size and simple design made it accessible to people of all ages and socioeconomic backgrounds, democratizing nail care practices and promoting better hygiene standards.

Before the Nail Clipper:

Before the invention of the nail clipper, people relied on a variety of tools and techniques to trim their nails. These included knives, scissors, and even specialized nail-cutting implements made of metal or bone. While effective to some extent, these tools were often crude and imprecise, posing a risk of injury or damage to the nails.

Nail hygiene

Why Cut Nails?

- Hygiene: Regularly trimming nails helps prevent the buildup of dirt, bacteria, and other microorganisms that can accumulate underneath the nails. This reduces the risk of infections and promotes overall hand and foot hygiene.
- Prevent Injury: Long nails can be prone to breakage, which can be painful and potentially lead to infections if the nail bed is damaged. Trimming nails to a moderate length helps prevent injuries and promotes nail health.
- Comfort: Overgrown nails, especially toenails, can cause discomfort and even pain when wearing shoes or engaging in physical activities. Trimming nails to a comfortable length can alleviate discomfort and improve mobility.
- Aesthetics: Well-groomed nails contribute to a neat and polished appearance. Trimming nails regularly helps maintain a tidy and professional look, whether at work, social events, or everyday activities.

How to Cut Nails:

Tools: Use proper nail care tools such as nail clippers or scissors specifically designed for cutting nails. Nail files can also be used to shape and smooth the edges after trimming.

Technique: Trim nails straight across to avoid ingrown nails, then gently round the edges with a nail file to prevent sharp corners. For toenails, avoid cutting them too short to reduce the risk of ingrown nails.

Frequency: It's recommended to trim fingernails and toenails regularly, approximately every 1-2 weeks, to maintain optimal nail health and hygiene.

Cleanliness: Wash hands and feet thoroughly before and after trimming nails to reduce the risk of infection. Ensure that nail care tools are clean and sanitized before use.

Biology of Nails:

Chemical Composition: Nails are primarily composed of a protein called keratin, which also makes up hair and the outer layer of skin. Keratin provides strength and structure to nails, helping to protect the delicate nail bed underneath.

Biological Function: Nails serve several biological functions, including protecting the fingertips and toes from trauma and providing tactile sensitivity. The nail plate, or visible part of the nail, helps enhance fingertip sensitivity and dexterity.

Sensory Perception: Unlike the skin, nails do not contain nerve endings, which is why they lack sensation. However, the surrounding nail bed and cuticle are sensitive to touch and pressure, providing sensory feedback to the fingertips.

Usage Habits and Cultural Significance:

Cultural Practices: Nail care practices vary widely across cultures and may hold symbolic or ritualistic significance. For example, in some cultures, long nails are associated with femininity or social status, while in others, short, well-groomed nails are preferred for practical reasons.

Personal Preferences: Individual preferences and habits also influence nail care routines. Some people enjoy experimenting with nail art and decorations, while others prefer a more minimalist approach to nail care.

Self-Care: Taking care of nails is not only about hygiene but also about self-care and personal grooming. Engaging in nail care rituals can be a form of self-expression and a way to pamper oneself.

Cutting fingernails and toenails is a simple yet important aspect of personal hygiene and grooming. By understanding the reasons behind nail care and adopting proper techniques, individuals can maintain healthy, well-groomed nails that contribute to overall well-being and confidence.

How to make clipping nails more fun?

How can we make the task of cutting nails more enjoyable turning it into a fun and creative activity than a painstaking chore? Here are 10 ways to make cutting nails more enjoyable:

1. Set the Mood: Create a relaxing atmosphere by playing your favorite music or lighting scented candles to make the experience more enjoyable and soothing.
2. Get Creative with Nail Art: Experiment with different nail art designs and techniques to add a fun and artistic flair to your nail care routine. Try out new colors, patterns, or even stickers to express your creativity.
3. Make it a Spa Day: Treat yourself to a mini spa day by soaking your hands or feet in warm water with essential oils or bath salts before trimming your nails. This can help soften the nails and cuticles, making the process more comfortable.
4. Try a DIY Manicure or Pedicure: Instead of just trimming your nails, give yourself a full DIY manicure or pedicure treatment. This can include shaping, buffing, and moisturizing your nails for a polished finish.
5. Invite a Friend: Turn nail care into a social activity by inviting a friend over for a nail care session. You can chat, laugh, and bond while pampering yourselves and sharing nail care tips and tricks.
6. Reward Yourself: Set up a reward system for yourself where you treat yourself to something you enjoy after completing your nail care routine. It could be a sweet treat, a relaxing bath, or even a new nail polish color to add to your collection.
7. Create a Nail Care Kit: Put together a personalized nail care kit with all your favorite tools, nail polishes, and accessories. Having everything you need in one place can make the process more organized and enjoyable.

8. Challenge Yourself: Set a nail care challenge for yourself, such as trying to master a new nail art technique or achieving a certain nail length. Challenge yourself to step out of your comfort zone and get creative with your nail care routine.
9. Host a Nail Art Party: Organize a nail art party with friends or family where everyone can bring their nail care supplies and get creative together. You can swap nail polish colors, share tips, and inspire each other with new nail art ideas.
10. Document Your Progress: Take photos of your nails before and after trimming them to track your progress over time. Seeing how your nails improve with regular care can be motivating and rewarding.

By incorporating these fun and creative ideas into your nail care routine, you can turn the task of cutting nails into a enjoyable and satisfying experience!

Nail-biting records

1. Lee Redmond: Lee Redmond from the United States held the Guinness World Record for the longest fingernails on a pair of hands until 2009. Her nails had a combined length of over 8.65 meters (28 feet 4.5 inches), with her longest nail, her right thumb, measuring 0.6 meters (2 feet). Redmond began growing her nails in 1979 and meticulously maintained them for decades. She protected her nails by avoiding activities that could damage them, such as washing dishes or household chores. Sadly, Redmond lost her record-setting nails in a car accident in 2009.
2. Ayanna Williams: Ayanna Williams, also from the United States, currently holds the record for the longest nails on a pair of hands. As of my last update, her nails measured over 7 meters (24 feet) in total length. Williams grew her nails over several decades, carefully protecting them and incorporating them into her daily life. She often wore gloves to protect her nails and adapted her daily routines to accommodate their length.
3. Chris Walton: Chris Walton, known as "The Dutchess," held the Guinness World Record for the longest fingernails on a pair of hands (female) until 2018. Her nails measured a combined length of over 8.65 meters (28 feet 4.5 inches). Walton grew her nails for over two decades, starting in the early 1990s. She often painted her nails with intricate designs and took special care to protect them from damage.
4. Shridhar Chillal: Shridhar Chillal from India held the record for the longest fingernails on a single hand until 2018. His thumbnail alone measured an astonishing 1.98 meters (6 feet 6 inches) in length. Chillal grew his nails for over six decades before finally deciding to cut them off in 2018. The nails were carefully removed during a ceremonial event in New York City and are now preserved in the Ripley's

Believe It or Not! Museum.

These individuals attracted worldwide attention for their remarkable nail growth and dedication to maintaining their record-setting nails. While their experiences varied, they all demonstrated extraordinary patience and commitment to their unique personal grooming habits. Cutting off their long nails marked the end of an era and garnered significant media coverage and public interest.

Anatomy of a fingernail

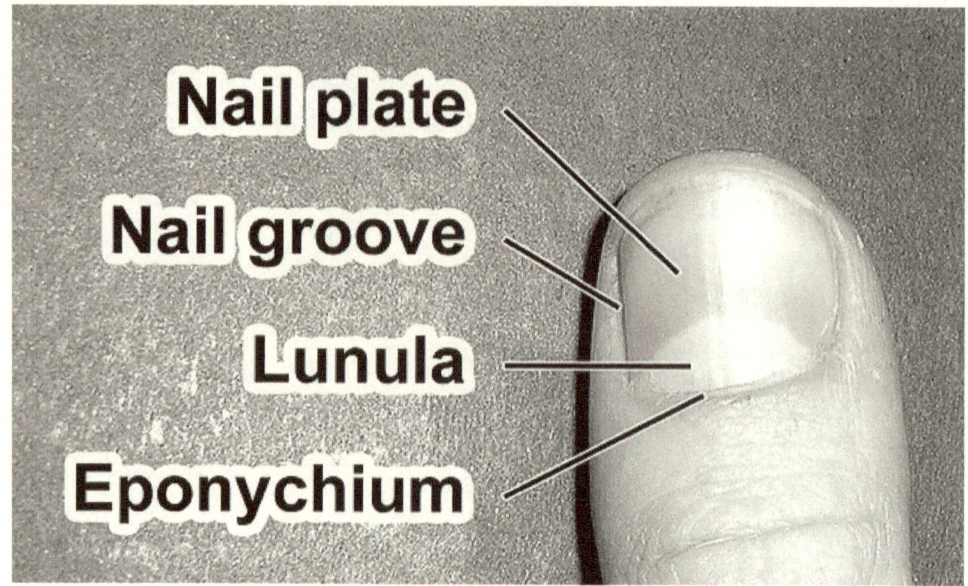

Frequency

The frequency of nail cutting varies from person to person and can depend on factors such as personal preference, lifestyle, and the rate of nail growth. However, as a general guideline:

1. Fingernails: Most people find that they need to trim their fingernails approximately every 1-2 weeks to maintain a neat and tidy appearance. Factors such as the rate of nail growth, daily activities, and personal grooming habits can influence how often fingernails need to be cut.

2. Toenails: Toenails typically grow at a slower rate than fingernails and may require less frequent trimming. On average, toenails may need to be cut every 3-4 weeks for most people. However,

individuals with faster-growing toenails or specific foot conditions may need to trim their toenails more frequently.

It's essential to pay attention to the length and condition of your nails to determine when they need to be trimmed. Long nails can be prone to breakage and may cause discomfort, while nails trimmed too short can lead to ingrown nails or irritation. Regular nail care, including trimming and shaping nails as needed, helps maintain nail health and promotes overall hygiene and aesthetics.

www.ingramcontent.com/pod-product-compliance
Lightning Source LLC
Chambersburg PA
CBHW051241250726
48656CB00003B/1064

* 9 7 9 8 3 2 3 2 0 1 2 4 2 *